Scrubs

ADISH Books

ISBN-13: 978-1492977414

ISBN-10: 1492977411

Text Copyright and Disclaimer © 2013 ADISH Books

ISBN-13: 978-1492977414

ISBN-10: 1492977411

Introduction - Natural Scrubs and Facial Masks

Exfoliating should be an important part of your skincare routine. It helps remove the buildup of dead cells from your face and body, and it contributes to great-looking skin. You will look visibly younger, and the health of your skin would improve as well.

After completing its life the cells of outer skin lay dead on the outer surface of the body. These dead cells should be naturally replaced by new cells from inner layer of the skin as designed by the nature. But due to our modern life style and polluted environment this natural process needs some outside help. We have to scrub or exfoliate these cells.

Regularly exfoliating your skin using natural and organic scrubs and masks ensures that the incidence of acne reduces. It improves blood circulation which increases the supply of nutrients and oxygen to the cells and this improves the health of cells. Exfoliation opens up clogged pores and lets your skin breathe freely. Exfoliation also ensures that cell renewal in your skin is fast and healthy.

While exfoliation is responsible for the health of your skin complexion, facials masks provide deep nourishment to the skin. It is very important to choose the correct mask for your skin type. Making your own facial masks at home using natural products give the face a spa-worth relaxation and rejuvenate the glow of the skin. You will look visibly younger, and the health of your skin would improve as well.

Why Use Organic Scrubs and Facial Masks?

Everything we put onto our body gets inside our body as well. It's all too easy to lather on a lotion containing toxic diethyl phthalate, giving little thought as to what effect it might have. However, studies conducted by the CDC show that these harsh chemicals make their way into the body. Although the effects of such substances are not fully known, one Harvard study showed a connection between concentrations of phthalates in the urine and DNA damage in human sperm. Other chemicals like sodium lauryl sulfate, petrochemicals, parabens, and formaldehyde releasing preservatives are common in cosmetic, beauty, and personal care products and are known to have cancer-causing effects. It makes you wonder...what other potentially dangerous chemicals do we expose ourselves to each day? What are the risks, and is there any benefit?

Natural and organic facial masks and body scrubs offer numerous benefits over non-natural options. The main reason for this is their ingredients. Normal scrubs and masks that are popular in the market and are often preferred over others come with inorganic and unnatural ingredients. By choosing non-natural facial masks and body scrubs, you expose your skin to the dangers of getting an allergy from chemicals.

Natural masks and scrubs have minimal to zero side effects. Many people experience skin irritations after using particular brands of scrubs and facial masks due to harsh chemical ingredients. However, these complaints are seldom heard with natural and organic scrubs and masks. Companies often try to replicate the effects of natural ingredients and use many chemical boosters and catalysts and our skin has to pay the price. Why use a substitute when you can use the real and natural thing? It would be much better for your skin if you treat it with the gentle care of natural ingredients

So stop exposing yourself to hundreds or even thousands of harsh chemicals. Natural products like Olive oil, Coconut oil, Almond oil and vitamin E oil work just as well as expensive, chemical-ridden products from the store. In many cases, natural products produce better results used on their own than in combination with chemical ingredients.

By using all-natural beauty products, you can save yourself time, money and prevent possible side effects. There's no reason to waste your money trying out dozens of products in order to find one that works for you. Go back to the basics. Try simple, all-natural products and get an all-natural, beautiful complexion in return.

The   Scrub

There are two different type of scrubs that can be used to exfoliate the skin. One is called a facial scrub, used specifically on the face. The other is called a body scrub and can be used generally on any part of the body.

Both facial and body scrubs are designed to exfoliate, removing dead skin and leaving it smooth, soft and hydrated. Scrubs are made with an abrasive ingredient like sugar, salt, rice bran or coffee grounds. They usually also contain a massage oil and essential oils to add a nice aroma. Some body scrubs are too harsh to use on soft, delicate facial skin. While a little exfoliation is good, too much can be harmful. Be careful not to use a harsh body scrub on your face. If a scrub is causing pain, stop using it.

You can enjoy a body or facial scrub in a spa.

Or, make or purchase your own scrub formula to use on your own at home. You shouldn't use a scrub every day. However, exfoliating your skin with a scrub once a week is a healthy practice.

It's easy to make your own scrub mix with a few common ingredients, and there are some benefits to making your own. Purchasing scrub formulas can get expensive fast. It's much more cost-effective to buy ingredients in bulk and whip them together when needed. It's also fun. With a few different oils and abrasives, you can make lots of unique combinations. They're fun and relaxing to use and make great gifts for friends and family members.

The Facial Mask

Although often overlooked, facial masks are an important step to any good skin care routine.

Although general cleansing routines work to rid your skin of dirt, oil and makeup, they're not always enough to completely cleanse your face.

Facial masks work deeper. They penetrate your pores, drawing out impurities and leaving cleaner, clearer skin. A face mask can be made out of ingredients like clay, fruit, mud, seaweed, algae, massage oils, vitamins, herbs, and essential oils. These ingredients are used to cleanse and hydrate the skin. They provide healthy vitamins, minerals and oils.

Different types of masks are used for different types of skin. Masks can also be used to treat various skin conditions like acne, eczema and acne scars. There are lots of benefits to using facial masks. They can tighten and tone the skin, draw out impurities like dirt and oil, heal blemishes and scarring, hydrate and nourish, and soothe irritated and inflamed skin.

There are different ways to apply masks. Some can be brushed onto the skin using a paint brush. Others can be applied by hand. They are removed by washing with warm water or a wet washcloth. Sometimes facial masks come with the ingredients already applied to a thin cloth or sheet in the shape of a mask. These are simply laid down and pressed against the face and then peeled off when finished. Masks using gel, latex or wax, often called peel off masks, can be peeled off by hand once dry.

A facial mask should generally be left on the skin for 10 to 15 minutes. For certain types of masks, the time may be increased or decreased. For peel off facials, the active ingredients take longer to set and should therefore be applied for longer than 15 minutes.

You can make your own mask right at home. All

you need are some natural, organic ingredients like honey, organic fruits and vegetables, milk, or egg whites. You can apply things like cucumbers and honey directly to your face. Or, mix several ingredients together to get more skin- healing benefits. Experimenting with homemade masks is fun and good for your skin!

Easily Available Natural Ingredients for Scrubs and Masks

The following are the most preferred natural scrubs and masks ingredients that are used for exfoliating purposes:

Aloe Vera – Aloe Vera has always been the miracle ingredient of skin care. It acts as an exfoliant by removing dead cells, and it leaves the skin baby soft to touch. Your skin would look smoother and brighter after you treat it with Aloe Vera. Also, Aloe Vera aids in the natural functions of the skin by helping retain moisture and boosting cell renewal. Even aging can be fought using Aloe Vera.

Almonds – For dry, sensitive skin, ground almonds act as an exfoliant and cleaner.

Avocado - Avocado contains high amounts of sterolins, which help reduce the appearance of scars, sun damage and age spots. It also helps heal eczema and dry skin. Avocado oil is also known to help increase the amount of collagen on the skin, slowing down the process of skin aging.

Olive Oil – People have been using olive oil for personal care for many centuries. It works great as a skin moisturizer as it contains linoleic acid, a compound that keeps the skin hydrated. It also contains at least four types of antioxidants, which help in neutralizing free radicals that lead to skin cancer and skin aging.

Baking Soda – Baking soda has a unique crystalline structure, which removes dead cells and works as an excellent exfoliant.

Coffee Bean – For dry skins that have a tendency to flake, ground coffee bean can be an effective exfoliant. It reduces dryness and exfoliates the flakes, and the result is a skin that feels softer.

Honey – Honey is another magic ingredient that improves the health of the skin in many ways. Using honey on the skin makes it fresh looking. It fights dry skin by keeping it hydrated. Honey also acts as a natural sun protection ingredient. It is antimicrobial in nature and has antioxidant properties that work in healing damaged skin by absorbing impurities that reside in skin pores. The skin is visibly smoother looking and feels silky soft after using honey.

Cornmeal – Choose the grain size depending on your skin type. Larger grains would be more abrasive than the finer ones. So, if you have acne, it is better to use finer grains to prevent scarring. Cornmeal scrubs make the skin soft, smooth and fresh.

Kelp – It is an unusual but highly effective ingredient that comes loaded with Vitamin A, Vitamin B complex, Vitamin C and Vitamin E. It also contains iodine and minerals that are excellent for the skin.

Sea Salt – Sea salt is used as a natural scrub, but the skin should not be damaged, dry or delicate. The texture of the salt is important and should not have jagged edges, which could harm the skin. The salt should feel smooth under your palm. After using sea salt, the skin would feel silky and dead cells would be removed, leaving the skin invigorated.

Caution While Exfoliating

Not all scrubs can be used for all skin types. Some scrubs work for all skin types while others are specific to a skin type. Skin prone to acne, acne rosacea and skin sensitive and thin in nature should be scrubbed very cautiously. Same goes for skin with broken capillaries. You could end up damaging your skin instead of making it better. Thus, care should be exercised.

A few instances exist when you should absolutely not use a facial scrub, natural or otherwise:

1. If your skin has been sunburned recently, then do not exfoliate your skin as your skin is already sensitive and is trying to heal.

2. Open cuts should not be scrubbed as the wound could get worst. Injured skin needs to be treated with gentle care and scrubbing would be too harsh.

3. Do not scrub and exfoliate skin that looks irritated. Get a doctor's opinion.

Know your Skin Type

It is very important to keep your skin type in mind while preparing scrub and mask. Most of the time people are confused about their skin type. Here are some simple characteristics to determine your skin type.

Normal / Combination Skin

Seventy percent of the total population all over the world has a normal or combination type of skin. This skin type is the least problematic and easy to maintain.

Characteristics:

- No traces of oil
- Vibrant, supple, and elastic
- Clean, smooth, and has good blood circulation
- Healthy and glowing complexion

How to determine

- It is slightly oily in the T-zone area of the face and the cheek areas are dry.
- Dry patchy spots are found anywhere in the body.
- Pores in the forehead and cheeks may be larger than the other parts of the face.

Oily Skin

This is the most problematic type of skin. Excessive oil on the skin may be caused by various changes, which may include hormonal changes, weather and temperature changes, and genetics.

Characteristics
- larger pores and break outs due to excessive oil in the face
- looks greasy, thick, and shiny
- prone to aging and wrinkle formation
- prone to blackheads, pimple, acne, and other skin blemishes

How to determine

- The T-zone of the face (from forehead, nose and chin) is shiny and greasy.
- It leaves oil marks or spots on a dermal paper.
- Excessive oil in the face even if the weather or temperature is fair.

Dry Skin

This type of skin requires special care. Most women experiences dry skin when they reached 35 years old. When exposed to drying factors, the skin cracks, peels, and becomes irritated and itchy. Dry skin may be caused by genetic factors, weather, aging, heat, medications, and application of skin care products.

Characteristics

- tight, dry, and scaly
- less elastic
- visible lines and pores

- red patches
- flaking

How to determine
- The dermal paper appears to be clean with a few oil spots.
- Upon washing the face, the skin feels tight, dry, and has a pale tone.

Sensitive Skin
This skin type is considered very fragile and requires a special type of skin care. It easily gets irritated to certain cosmetic products.

Characteristics
- thin and delicate
- fine pores

How to determine
- If a cosmetic product is not suitable for the

skin, it results to itching, dryness, redness, and even burning of the skin.

Scrub Recipes by Skin Type

Scrubs for Normal/Combination Skin

Rejuvenating Rosemary Lavender Salt Scrub

Ingredients:

- 2 cups of salt

- 3 tablespoons of lavender

- ¼ cup of olive oil

- 3 tablespoons of finely chopped rosemary leaves

- 1 bowl for mixing

Instructions:

- In a bowl, mix the salt and the olive oil. Mix well.

- Add in the chopped rosemary leaves and the lavender. Blend all ingredients thoroughly.

Benefits: The olive oil ingredient of this scrub is rich in fatty acid, which can efficiently hold moisture on the skin without drying the skin out. Moreover, rosemary leaves are also beneficial since these have potent rejuvenation ability. These improve blood circulation and skin complexion, giving the skin a healthy pink glow. Lavender contains relaxing effects, which helps revitalize stressed skin.

Invigorating Peppermint Sugar Scrub

Ingredients:

- 2 cups of white granulated sugar

- 10 drops of peppermint essential oil

- ¼ cup of coconut oil or almond oil

- Raspberry or pomegranate juice

- 1 bowl for mixing

Instructions:

- In a mixing bowl, combine coconut oil or almond oil with granulated sugar. Check mixture and add ingredients liberally. However, make sure that the mixture will not get too oily.

- Add in the peppermint essential oil until the desired scent is achieved.

- To achieve the pink color of the scrub, add in a few drops of pomegranate juice or raspberry juice.

- Mix all ingredients thoroughly and make sure that the color is uniform.

Benefits: The peppermint ingredient will help you feel refreshed and invigorated. This also helps soothe as well as heal the skin. This can efficiently nourish and hydrates the skin. The Coconut oil or almond oil has moisturizing properties that keep the skin hydrated. Raspberry juice helps detoxify and renews aging skin.

Renewing Pineapple Scrub

Ingredients:

- 2/3 cup of fresh pineapple chunks

- ¼ cup fresh and finely chopped parsley

- ¼ cup olive oil

- Blender

Instructions:

- Place pineapple chunks in the blender and press on pulse.

- Add in olive oil until the mixture is smooth.

- Add the parsley and blend mixture thoroughly and avoid liquefying the mixture.

Benefits: The pineapple ingredient of this scrub has natural chemicals that will help dissolve the bonds that hold the skin cells together. Once dissolved, dead skin cells will slough off easily, which makes way for healthy new skin cells. Parsley works great for treating and preventing acne as it is a natural antiseptic. Olive oil also contains oleic acid that helps soften the skin and vitamin E that helps improve the skin's elasticity.

Moisturizing Oatmeal and Lavender Scrub

Ingredients:

- 1 cup of ground oatmeal

- ½ cup of powdered milk

- ½ cup dry lavender flowers

- 2 teaspoon of cornmeal

- 1 bowl for mixing

Instructions:

- In a bowl, mix the ground oatmeal with the powdered milk. Mix well.

- Add in the dry lavender flowers with the cornmeal. Blend all ingredients thoroughly.

Benefits: The oatmeal and cornmeal ingredients of this scrub are most beneficial for normal skin as this comes with exfoliating, cleansing, and moisturizing properties. This scrub will leave the skin looking smooth, soft, radiant, and healthy. Milk contains fatty acids that moisturize the skin. Lavender flowers provide soothing effects that help relax the skin.

Sunless Tanner Scrub

Ingredients:

- 5 cups of white granulated sugar

- 2 cups of olive oil

- 3 tablespoons honey

- 2 lemons

- 1 mixing bowl

Instructions:

- In a bowl, combine sugar and olive oil.

- Slice the lemons in half and squeeze its juice into the sugar and olive oil mixture.

- Add honey into the mixture and combine thoroughly.

Benefits: This scrub is great for healthy exfoliation of the normal skin types due to the citric acid from lemons. Citric acid is a natural exfoliating substance, and this ingredient causes bleaching, which is a great sunless tanner. Olive oil contains fatty acids that help keep the skin hydrated. The antiseptic properties of honey helps prevent and treat skin blemishes.

Pineapple and Aloe Vera Facial Scrub

Ingredients:

- 2/3 cup pineapple chunks

- ¼ cup Aloe Vera juice (slime)

- ¼ cup chopped parsley

- ¼ cup olive oil

Instructions:

- In a blender, slightly blend the pineapple chunks.

- Pour olive oil to the pineapple in the blender and then, blend until it is almost smooth.

- Include parsley to the mixture and then, blend without turning it into a liquid texture.

Benefits: This scrub can give smoother, younger skin. Pineapple and Aloe Vera, which is rich in alpha-hydroxy acids, can naturally exfoliate skin to get rid of the dead skin layers. Parsley, which is rich in Vitamin C, can cleanse pores and reduce fine lines.

Refreshing Lime and Honey Facial Scrub

Ingredients:

- 1/3 cup nuts (unsalted)

- 1/3 cup oats (rolled)

- 1 tbsp honey

- 1 tbsp grapeseed oil

- ¼ cup milk

- ½ lime juice

Instructions:

- Mix nuts and oats. Grind them to a fine, powdery finish with the use of a food processor.

- Include the rest of the ingredients. Mix thoroughly. This should have a thin consistency. If not, more milk should be added.

Benefits: Oats absorb excess oil in the face, leaving it clean. Honey and grapeseed oil contains hydrating properties that help preserve moisture in the skin while nuts make face supple. This invigorating scrub makes skin look and feel refreshed.

Calming Lavender, Vanilla and Honey Face Scrub

Ingredients:

- 1 tablespoon honey

- 1 teaspoon almond oil (can be replaced with jojoba or grapeseed oil)

- 1 teaspoon pure vanilla extract

- 1 teaspoon dried lavender

- ¼ cup light brown sugar

- ¼ cup white sugar

Instructions:

- Wisk white and brown sugar together in a bowl.

- Stir in vanilla in the sugar mixture until evenly distributed.

- Add lavender into the mixture, crushing the buds gently between your fingers.

- Stir in the oil and honey, mixing until the mixture is even and a thick consistency is reached.

- Transfer the mixture in an air-tight container and label appropriately.

Benefits: Lavender and vanilla have calming properties. Honey absorbs impurities and detoxifies the skin. It is a great moisturizer, which leaves the face feeling extra soft. This simple face scrub can give clearer, blemish-free skin.

Wheat Flour and Extra Virgin Olive Oil Face Scrub

Ingredients:

- 1 tbsp wheat flour

- 1 tsp extra virgin olive oil

- ½ tsp turmeric

- ½ tsp lemon juice

Instructions:

- Mix all ingredients thoroughly in a bowl then make it into a paste.

Benefits: Wheat flour has vitamin E that slows down aging. Turmeric is rich in antioxidants that can give a more youthful skin. It can also reduce pigmentation to even out skin tone. Lemon juice can tighten pores, eliminate excess oil, and help lighten skin, which will eventually fade away dark spots and freckles.

Detoxifying Green Tea Face Scrub

Ingredients:

- 3 tsp green tea

- 2 tsp brown sugar

- 1 tsp nourishing cream

Instructions:

- Mix all the ingredients in a bowl and make into a paste.

Benefits: This scrub is suitable for combination skin because of its potent ingredient, green tea. This powerful antioxidant can reduce water retention or puffiness in the face. It also calms down redness, detoxifies facial skin pores, and reduces inflammation caused by acne breakouts. Brown sugar is an ideal exfoliator because of its texture. It removes dead skin cells to pave the way for smoother, supple skin.

Scrub Recipes for Dry Skin

Nourishing Avocado and Ground Almond Scrub

Ingredients:

- 1 avocado, medium ripe, peeled, and mashed

- 1 cup ground oatmeal

- 1/3 cup ground almonds or ground hazelnuts

Instructions:

- In a bowl, mix the mashed avocado with the ground almonds or hazelnuts. Mix these ingredients thoroughly.

- Add in the ground oatmeal in the mixture and mix well.

Optional: Adding ½ cup dried lavender to the mixture provides a calming effect to the skin.

Benefits: Avocado contains vitamin A that softens and repairs the skin. Also, the fatty acids found in almonds help keep the skin hydrated and nourished. Oatmeal's cleansing properties helps exfoliate dry skin easily. This buttery scrub is beneficial as this can moisturize dry skin types while nourishing it.

Hydrating Coffee Scrub

Ingredients:

- 1/4 cup of olive oil

- 1 cup of brown sugar

- ½ cup of used coffee grounds which is from a freshly brewed pot

- 1 teaspoon of pure vanilla extract

- 15 drops of peppermint essential oil

Instructions:

- In a bowl, mix the ¼ cup of olive oil and the brown sugar. Mix these ingredients thoroughly.

- Add the pure vanilla extract before adding 15 drops of the peppermint essential oil.

- Once thoroughly blended together, add in the ground coffee. Make sure all ingredients are blended together.

Optional: Adding Tea Tree oil extract to the mixture can add healing effects for acne prone dry skin.

Benefits: This scrub can help cleanse as well as soften dry skin. Coffee is effective in promoting moisture retention, which is beneficial for those people with dry skin. Olive oil is also rich in monounsaturated fats and polyphenols, which provide deep moisturizing effect on the skin. This scrub will definitely leave your skin softer, smoother and more radiant.

Ingredients:

- 1 ½ cup brown sugar

- 1 tablespoon jojoba oil or sweet almond oil

- 1 cup coconut oil

- Pink or red rose petals

- 1 clean jar with a lid

Instructions:

- This scrub should be prepared a few days before this is used.

- To start off, pour the coconut oil into the jar with the lid.

- Add in the pink or red rose petals into the jar.

- Then, add in the raw sugar and the jojoba oil or sweet almond oil.

- Once all ingredients are placed inside the jar, mash them together using a large spoon.

Benefits: The jojoba oil is an effective moisturizer. This essential oil can be easily absorbed by the skin, which leaves dry skin feeling soft and supple. The rose petals also have natural oils, which help lock in moisture on dry skin and making it soft.

Olive Oil Scrub for Moisturizing and Repairing

Ingredients:

- ½ cup sea salt

- ¼ cup olive oil

- ½ cup brown sugar

- 15 drops of orange essential oil

Instructions:

- In a bowl, mix brown sugar and the sea salt thoroughly.

- Then, add in the olive oil. Mix these ingredients well before adding in 15 drops of orange essential oil.

Benefits: The olive oil ingredient helps dry skin by regaining its natural oil balance, and this can effectively repair dry skin while keeping it soft and smooth. Sea salt is known to have high concentration of magnesium that promotes skin hydration and reduces inflammation. Orange essential oil also contains healing properties that help correct skin imbalance.

Moisturizing Citrus Scrub

Ingredients:

- 1 cup of sea salt

- 1 cup of olive oil

- 1 tablespoon of lemon zest

- 2 drops of grapefruit essential oil

- 1 jar with lid

Instructions:

- In a lidded jar, pour in the sea salt and olive oil and mix well.

- Add in the lemon zest and the grapefruit essential oil. Combine all ingredients thoroughly.

Benefits: Grapefruit contains properties that can help in exfoliating dry skin while olive oil helps lock in moisture and smoothness on the skin.

Scrubs for Oily Skin

Sugar and Olive Oil Scrub for Oil Reduction and Repair

Ingredients:

- 1 tablespoon of sugar

- 1 tablespoon of virgin olive oil (preferably extra virgin olive oil)

- 1 medium sized container or jar

Instructions:

- In a medium-sized container, put 1 tablespoon of sugar and 1 table spoon of extra virgin olive oil.

- Mix the two ingredients well until a paste-like consistency is achieved.

Benefits:

Extra virgin coconut oil contains numerous minerals and vitamins that can make skin smooth and oil free. The natural substance in this oil is also known to soften, moisturize, and heal damaged skin. Sugar is a natural exfoliant and helps in reducing excess oil on the skin.

Lightening Honey and Almonds Scrub

Ingredients:

- Almonds

- 2 tablespoon of honey

- 1 medium sized container or jar

Instructions:

- Place a handful of almonds in a container and make a powder.

- Add 2 tablespoons of honey and mix it thoroughly with the almonds.

Benefits: Almonds are identified to be a great lightening material that can help reduce blemishes and other skin marks. Moreover, almonds have anti-oxidant properties and are rich in Vitamin E. Honey is a very good moisturizer and agent to keep the skin soft and smooth.

Revitalizing Sea Salt and Lemon Juice Scrub

Ingredients:

- 1 ½ tablespoons of lemon juice

- 1 tablespoon of sea salt

- 1 medium sized container or jar

Instructions:

- Put 1 ½ tablespoons of lemon juice and 1 tablespoon of sea salt in a container.

- Mix the two ingredients thoroughly.

Benefits: Lemon juice aids in reducing the marks and blemishes on the skin. Sea salt is the best agent for scrubbing the skin since it has a high mineral content that can help remove excess oil. Furthermore, sea salt has as numerous benefits on the skin including moisturizing, exfoliating, revitalizing, and cleansing.

Sea Salt, Egg, and Lime Juice Scrub

Ingredients:

- 1 egg white

- 2 tablespoons of sea salt

- ½ tablespoon of lime juice

- 1 medium sized container or jar

Instructions:

- In a container, put 1 egg white, 2 tablespoons of sea salt, and ½ tablespoon of lime juice.

- Mix all the ingredients thoroughly.

Benefits:

Egg white helps assist in making the skin tight while the lime juice aids in skin lightening, softening, and reducing the blemishes.

Furthermore, aside from moisturizing the skin, sea salt's antiseptic properties also helps in removing excess oil, germs, and bacteria on the skin.

Oats, Strawberry, and Lemon Juice Scrub

Ingredients:

- 2 to 3 ripe strawberry

- 2 tablespoons of oatmeal

- ½ tablespoon of lemon juice

- 1 medium sized container or jar

Instructions:

- Mash 2 to 3 strawberries.

- Grind the oats.

- Put the mashed strawberries and grinded oats in a container.

- Add the lemon juice.

- Mix all the ingredients thoroughly.

Benefits: Strawberry has an acidic property that can help remove oil on skin and take away all dead skin cells. It also has salicylic acid that can help fight acne and blackheads. Oatmeal has properties that can heal and nourish skin. It is hypoallergenic and has amino acids that can help keep the skin hydrated.

Scrub Recipes for Sensitive Skin

Energizing Citrus Salt Scrub

Ingredients:

- 16 tablespoons of olive oil

- 16 tablespoons of sea salt

- 1 tablespoon of lemon or citrus

- 2 drops of any essential oil (Lavender, grapefruit, rose)

Instructions:

- Mix all the ingredients in a bowl until the mixture is completely thick.

- Pour the mixture into a jar with a tight cover or any preferred container.

- Label the jar or container according to use.

Benefits: The citrus or lemon contains vitamin C that energizes the skin from stress and can whiten the skin as well. The salt serves as a pore cleanser and helps in removing dead skin cells. Olive oil gives moisture and makes the skin feeling smooth and silky.

Moisturizing Rose Petal and Sugar Scrub

Ingredients:

- 32 tablespoons of turbinado brown sugar

- 16 tablespoons of virgin coconut oil

- 1 tablespoon of any essential oil (jojoba oil or sweet almond)

- Petals from a rose

- 1 big jar

Instructions:

- In a large kind of jar, pour the virgin coconut oil and a handful amount of rose petals.

- Add the brown sugar and essential oil on top of the petals.

- With a use of a spoon, mash the ingredients together until the mixture is thick and even.

- Cover the jar tightly or transfer the scrub into a preferred container.

Benefits: The brown sugar exfoliates the dead skin cells while the virgin coconut oil moisturizes the skin. The rose petal has antioxidant properties that help delay the aging of the skin cells.

Energizing Coffee and Turbinado Brown Sugar Scrub

Ingredients:

- 4 tablespoons of olive oil

- 16 tablespoons of turbinado brown sugar

- . 75 ml of peppermint essential oil

- 8 tablespoons of ground coffee from a newly brewed coffee

Instructions:

- Add all the ingredients in a large bowl and mix thoroughly.

- Make sure that the brown sugar and ground coffee is mixed evenly to form scrub granules.

- Pour the coffee scrub into a jar or any container and label according to use.

Benefits: The awakening coffee scrub revitalizes the tired skin from stress and at the same time nourishes it from severe damage. The brown sugar deeply exfoliates the skin along with the ground coffee, which also serves as a natural antioxidant agent. The peppermint essential oil's rejuvenating properties awaken and energize the skin, making it more radiant and beautiful.

Intense Nourishing Avocado and Nut Scrub

Ingredients:

- 1 piece of ripe avocado fruit (medium sized)

- 5 tablespoons of ground nuts (almond or hazelnut)

- 16 tablespoons of refined oatmeal

Instructions:

- Peel the medium sized avocado and mash it in a small bowl.

- In a larger bowl, mix the mashed avocado fruit, ground nuts, and refined oatmeal.

- Mix all the ingredients until consistency is thick and even.

- Pour the scrub in a jar or any container and cover tightly.

- Label as needed or according to use.

Benefits: The oats and nuts are rich in essential fatty acids that help exfoliate the dead skin cells, allowing new skin cells to form. The avocado butter's hydrating properties help moisturize and nourish the skin, keeping it smooth with a youthful glow.

Revitalizing and Nourishing Olive Oil and Sugar Scrub

Ingredients:

- 8 tablespoons of Epson Salt

- 8 tablespoons of demarara brown sugar

- 4 cups of olive oil

- 2 drops of any citrus essential oil

Instructions:

- Mix the Epsom salt, brown sugar, and olive oil in a bowl.

- After mixing the ingredients thoroughly, add the essential oil and stir to blend.

- Pour the scrub into a container and cover properly.

Benefits: The Epson salt and demarara brown sugar are natural exfoliants that help remove the dead skin cells. The citrus essential oil helps energize the skin from stress. Olive oil contains hydrating properties that deeply moisturize and nourish the skin.

Natural Face Mask Recipes by Skin Type

Here are the facial masks recipes for different skin types and its corresponding skin benefits.

Face Masks for Normal/ Combination Skin

Turmeric Mask for Healing and Toning

Ingredients:

- 2 tsp. turmeric powder

- 2 tsp. almond oil

- 2 tsp. sandalwood powder

- ½ cup besan

Instructions:

Combine all the ingredients. Add some oil then mix to make a paste.

Benefits: Turmeric is used to counteract skin imbalances by reducing pimples and spots in the face. It also hydrates the skin. It adds color to pale skin, giving a radiant glow to the complexion. It is a powerful anti-oxidant and has anti-microbial and anti-inflammatory properties. Almond oil makes skin supple. Sandalwood, with its antimicrobial properties, soothes the skin and fades away blemishes, spots, and scars. Also, it tones skin and lightens complexion.

Revitalizing and Nourishing Peach Mask

Ingredients:

- 1 peach

- 1 tbsp. oatmeal

- 1 tbsp. honey

Instructions:

- Cook the peach until it is very soft, and then mash it with a spoon.

- Add oatmeal and honey until it forms a thick and consistent paste.

Benefits: Peaches let people have young and refreshing skin. They do wonders for tired skin, enabling it to regain its luster. A peach is loaded with vitamins that nourish and brighten the skin's complexion. It also tightens pores.

Oatmeal is known to absorb oil and exfoliate dead skin cells. Honey has anti-microbial properties and contains antioxidants, which help skin look younger.

Rejuvenating Papaya and Honey Mask

Ingredients:

- ½ cup of papaya

- 2 tbsp. honey

Instructions:

- Mash the papaya in the bowl.

- Blend the honey with the papaya.

Benefits: Papaya is rich in vitamins and antioxidants that give a healthy, beautiful skin. It consists of rejuvenating enzymes that allow it to exfoliate the skin. It gets rid of the dead skin cells so that a new, radiant skin will surface. This cleanses and refreshes tired looking skin. Honey has long been used as a skin enhancer by most people. It has antioxidants that give a more youthful skin. It is also a good exfoliant.

Nourishing Carrot and Parsley Mask

Ingredients:

- ¼ cup carrot juice

- 1 tsp. parsley

- ¼ cup white clay

Instructions:

Combine all the ingredients together to create a creamy mask.

Benefits: A carrot has qualities that help tone the skin. It can cleanse and detoxify the skin to get rid of its impurities without causing any irritation or drying it. It prevents discoloration and the signs of aging. Parsley is rich in vitamin C, which allows it to speed up the production of collagen. It can cleanse pores and regulate production of oil. It nourishes the skin to reduce fine lines.

Lightening Marie Antoinette Mask

Ingredients:

- 1 egg

- 1 lemon

- 1 tbsp. witch hazel

- 4 tbsp. non-fat milk powder (dry)

Instructions:

Use a blender in mixing all of the ingredients.

Benefits: Witch hazel has anti-inflammatory properties, which are used as an anti-aging skin treatment. It has anti-microbial properties that can prevent microbial skin conditions. Furthermore, it is considered as a potent astringent and moisturizer. Lemon gets rid of pigmentation and dark spots. Its juice is effective in treating acne and in removing blackheads. This can also lighten the skin and helps get rid of acne marks. The carotenoid antioxidant present in eggs preserves the skin's elasticity.

Green Clay Mask

Ingredients:

- 1 ½ teaspoon green clay

- 1 ½ teaspoon aloe vera gel

- ½ teaspoon kaolin clay

- 2 drops of rose essential oil

- 1 tablespoon rosewater

- 1 mixing bowl

Instructions:

- In a mixing bowl, combine the green clay and the kaolin clay. Mix the two ingredients well.

- Add the aloe vera gel into the mixture and combine thoroughly.

- Combine the rosewater and the rose essential oil into the mixture.

- Refrigerate the mixture up to four weeks.

Benefits: Kaolin clay helps purify, soothe, nourish, and heal different skin types. This is an ideal ingredient in facial masks since this is chemical free. It contains essential enzymes that help improve blood circulation in the skin, eliminating toxins and wastes. Aloe vera, on the other hand, has a soothing and smoothing effect on the skin.

Reviving Cocoa and Coffee Skin Mask

Ingredients:

- 4 tablespoons of finely ground coffee beans

- 4 tablespoons of unsweetened cocoa powder

- 8 tablespoons of dairy product whole milk, heavy cream, almond milk, yogurt or coconut milk

- 2 tablespoons of honey or lemon juice

- 1 mixing bowl

Instructions:

- Combine the ground coffee beans and the cocoa powder in a mixing bowl.

- Stir in the dairy product to the mixture. Stir the ingredients well until the mixture turns into a smooth paste form. Lesser dairy product may be used if you would like to achieve a thicker paste.

- Add honey or lemon juice. You can use lemon juice if you have an oily skin or honey if you have a dry skin.

Benefits: The combination of coffee and cocoa can decrease the puffiness of the face especially in the eye area. This combination can also help brighten the skin and improve skin complexion. Honey is an effective moisturizer and contains anti aging properties. Lemon juice brightens the skin's complexion and revives dull looking skin.

Moisturizing Yogurt and Oatmeal Face Mask

Ingredients:

- 1 tablespoon of finely ground oatmeal

- 1 tablespoon of unflavored organic yogurt

- 5 drops of honey

- 1 mixing bowl

Instructions:

- In a mixing bowl, combine the ground oatmeal and yogurt. Mix the two ingredients together.

- Separately, warm 5 drops of honey. To be able do this, place a spoon under hot water for several minutes. Once warm, add in the honey on the spoon.

- Stir the warm honey into the oatmeal and yogurt mixture.

Benefits: This facial mask can cleanse as well as rejuvenate the skin. Oatmeal has moisturizing properties. It also has cleansing and exfoliating properties which are perfect for any skin types. Yogurt and honey contains anti-oxidant, keeping the skin free from blemishes and spots.

Soothing Yogurt and Egg White Face Mask

Ingredients:

- 2 egg whites

- 2 tablespoons plain yogurt

- 1 mixing bowl

Instructions:

- Place the egg whites in a mixing bowl. Make sure to separate the yolk from the egg whites.

- Add in the yogurt and mix the ingredients well.

Benefits: This facial mask is rather easy to make and this is beneficial for all skin types. This can help in effectively moisturizing as well as soothing the skin. Egg whites can tighten skin pores while providing a natural face lift. Yogurt, on the other hand, is an effective ingredient that makes   the   skin   smooth.

Rejuvenating Pumpkin Mask

Ingredients:

- 2 eggs

- ½ cup of fresh pumpkin pulp

- 2 teaspoons of almond milk for dry skin

- 1 teaspoon of honey for dry skin

- 2 teaspoons of cranberry juice or apple cider vinegar for oily skin

Instructions:

- Puree the pumpkin pulp until it turns into a thick paste.

- Combine the eggs into the puree.

- Combine almond milk and honey into the mixture if you have dry skin. For oily skin, skip the almond milk and honey. Stir in the cranberry juice or the apple vinegar cider instead.

- Mix the ingredients well.

Benefits: Pumpkin is rich in natural exfoliating acids as well as antioxidants, which help brighten and soften the skin. Eggs contain properties that help lock-in moisture, keeping the skin hydrated. Honey and apple cider vinegar have antiseptic properties that help prevent breakouts.

Face Masks for Dry Skin

Moisturizing Avocado Mask

Ingredients:

- ½ ripe avocado

- 1 tbsp. olive oil

- 1 tbsp. lemon juice

- 1 egg white

- 1 tbsp. honey

Instructions:

- Place the avocado in a bowl. Mash it with a fork.

- Add olive oil and lemon juice. Mix it well.

- Add egg white and mix.

- Add honey and mix.

Benefits: This mask soothes hydrates and moisturizes the skin. When applied topically, avocado can hydrate parched skin. Olive oil is a natural moisturizer. Lemon is a natural exfoliant, which removes dead skin, leaving it smooth and soft. Egg white tightens skin. Honey has mild alpha hydroxyl acids that make it a great exfoliant.

Hydrating and Soothing Cucumber and Aloe Mask

Ingredients:

- 1 pc. Cucumber

- 2 tbsp. aloe vera

Instructions:

- Peel the cucumber and remove all its seeds.

- Slice the cucumber into tiny pieces then place them in a food processor.

- Add aloe vera.

- Blend until mixture turns into a smooth paste.

Benefits: This mask gives tones the skin to make it look more radiant. Cucumber is soothing due to its nutrients and phytochemicals. It is a great source of hydration, which is needed for a glowing complexion. It contains silica, which reduces fine lines. Aloe vera soothes dry skin and prevents cracking.

Repairing and Moisturizing Banana and Yogurt Mask

Ingredients:

- ½ banana

- 4 tbsps. plain yogurt

Instructions:

- Place the banana in a small bowl then mash it with a fork.

- Add yogurt to the mashed banana then stir until the mixture is very smooth.

Benefits: This mask can add a glow to dry skin, making it look for fresh and youthful. A banana has vitamin A, which restores lost moisture and repairs damaged skin. It is rich in vitamin C, which maintains the skin's youthful glow.

Yogurt has lactic acid, which softens, tightens, and refines the skin pores. It has anti-bacterial properties that get rid of germs.

Protecting and Moisturizing Carrot and Avocado Mask

Ingredients:

- 1 pc. carrot (peeled)

- 1 tbsp. honey

- ½ avocado

- ½ tbsp. extra virgin olive oil

- 1 tsp. lemon juice

- 1 egg yolk

Instructions:

- Boil or steam the carrot until tender. Then mash it with a form until it becomes creamy.

- Mash the avocado together with the carrot.

- Include lemon juice, honey and egg yolk.

Benefits: This mask deeply moisturizes facial skin. Carrots are rich in vitamin A and anti-oxidants that protect skin against sun damage. Avocados hydrate dry skin. Egg yolks have omega-6 fatty acids that help maintain healthy skin.

Hydrating Orange Face Mask

Ingredients:

- 3 pcs. orange peel

- Milk

Instructions:

- Peel the oranges with the use of a grater. Leave the orange zest in bowl for about 1 to 2 days until dry.

- Place dried orange zest in a blender. Blend until this turns into powder.

- Combine powder with an equal amount of milk until it forms a paste.

Benefits: This mask makes skin more hydrated to prevent wrinkles. Orange has moderate acidity that has astringent properties. When combined with the right ingredient, it can help rebuild collagen. Milk balances the skin's pH. It regenerates and tones the skin.

Face Masks for Oily Skin

Gentle Oatmeal Mask

Ingredients:

- Oatmeal

- 1 tbsp. honey

- 1 egg yolk

Instructions:

- Combine egg yolk and honey in a bowl.

- Gradually add just enough oatmeal to make a thick paste.

Benefits: This mask will leave your face fresh and shine free. When oatmeal is applied to the skin, it is capable of absorbing excess oils, effectively treating oily skin and reducing blemishes. Honey has humectant properties that moisturize skin without making it too oily. It has antibacterial properties, which can help fight acne and absorb impurities from skin pores. The egg yolk helps retain skin moisture.

Strawberry, Honey, Brown Sugar Mask

Ingredients:

- 6 strawberries (without stem)

- 1 tbsp. honey

- 1 tbsp. brown sugar

- 1 tbsp. lemon juice

Instructions:

- Place strawberries in a food processor.

- Add honey, brown sugar and lemon juice. Blend in food processor to make a paste.

Benefits: Strawberries have salicylic acid, which can treat acne, skin discoloration, wrinkles, and sun damage. Brown sugar is a natural exfoliant. Honey has antiseptic properties that allow it to absorb excess oil and eliminate acne. Lemon juice is a great toner for oily skin. It is effective in addressing acne and inflammation in the skin.

Green Clay Mask

Ingredients:

- 1 tbsp. green clay

- 3 drops palmarosa essential oil

- 1 tsp. apricot kernel oil

Instructions:

- Combine palmarosa essential oil and apricot kernel oil.

- Add some drops of warm water then mix. Add some more water when necessary to make a spreadable paste.

Benefits: This is a purifying mask. Green clay is mineral clay, which cleans pores and absorbs excess oil. It has the ability to exfoliate. So it can remove dead skin cells and prevent blemishes to give a clearer skin. Palmarosa essential oil regulates skin moisture while apricot kernel oil is a gentle moisturizer.

Revitalizing Plum and Yogurt Mask

Ingredients:

- 4 plums

- 2 tbsp. plain yogurt

- 1 tsp. sweet almond oil

- Corn flour

Instructions:

- Poach the plums then strain well. Leave them to cool.

- Mash the plums then add yogurt and sweet almond oil.

- Add some corn flour to thicken.

Benefits: This is for oily skin that is prone to spots. Plum is rich in antioxidants like Vitamin

A and C. These can help in controlling oil and preventing acne. Yogurt has lactic acid, which helps in shedding dead skin cells. Sweet almond oil contains anti-microbial properties that prevent spread of bacteria.

Carrot Mask for Toning

Ingredients:

- 1 large carrot

- 1 tbsp. honey

- 1 tbsp. yogurt

Instructions:

- Boil the carrot then mash it. This can be done with a food processor.

- Add honey and yogurt.

Benefits: Since carrots are rich in vitamin A, they make a great mask to treat acne scars and blemishes, which are more common in oily skin. Honey has anti-microbial properties that prevent the growth of acne-causing bacteria. Its humectant properties let skin remain supple. It has the ability to remove dead skin cells on the skin's outer surface. Yogurt makes a good skin toner.

Face Masks for Sensitive Skin

Egg White, Cucumber and Avocado Facial Mask

Ingredients:

- 8 tablespoons of chopped cucumber

- 8 tablespoons of chopped avocado

- 1 piece of raw egg

- ½ tablespoon of powdered milk

Instructions:

- Break the egg and separate the yolk and the egg white.

- In a blender, pour the chopped cucumber, chopped avocado, and powdered milk.

- Blend the ingredients until the consistency is smooth, thick and paste like.

- Add the egg white into the mixture and blend it thoroughly.

- Pour the mixture into a container and label properly.

Benefits: This revitalizing facial mask cleanses, moisturizes, nourishes, and whitens the skin. The cucumber regenerates the skin cells and at the same time deeply cleanses the skin. The avocado fruit nourishes and serves as an antioxidant agent that delays skin aging. The egg white fights acne and improves the skin tone and texture. Milk contains properties that nourish sensitive skin, making it younger looking and radiant.

Avocado and Lemon Quencher Moisturizing Mask

Ingredients:

- 1 piece of ripe avocado

- ½ tablespoon of lemon juice

- ½ tablespoon of avocado

Instructions:

- Peel the avocado and remove the seed.

- Puree the flesh of the avocado fruit until it is moist and soft.

- Add the avocado oil and lemon juice and stir thoroughly.

- Mix the ingredients until the consistency is thick and paste like.

- Pour into a container and label properly.

Benefits: The Avocado and Lemon Quencher face mask revitalizes the sensitive skin with its avocado and lemon ingredients. The avocado nourishes and moisturizes the skin. The lemon removes scar and lightens the dark spots. This facial mask is recommended for sensitive skin because of its natural ingredients.

Homey Banana Peeling Face Mask

Ingredients:

- 1 piece of ripe banana

- ½ tablespoon of honey

- ½ tablespoon of lemon juice

Instructions:

- Peel the ripe banana and put it in a bowl.

- With the use of fork, mash the banana until the mixture is soggy and paste like.

- Add the lemon juice and honey.

- Mix thoroughly until the mixture is thick and even.

- Pour into a container and label according to use.

Benefits: This facial mask is perfect for a sensitive skin with problems of acne and infection. The honey moisturizes and traps dirt that is deeply located in the pores. The banana on the other hand, serves as antibacterial agent and cleanser that thoroughly cleanse the skin. The lemon tones and lightens the dark spots when the acne is removed.

Lemon Green Juice Facial Mask for Healing

Ingredients:

- 1 piece of fresh raw egg

- 3- 5 drops of lemon juice

Instructions:

- Break the egg and separate the yolk from the egg white. Preserve or discard the egg yolk.

- In a separate bowl, whisk the egg white until the mixture is foamy.

- Add the drops of lemon and mix until the mixture is even.

- Pour the mixture into a container and label according to use.

Benefits: This facial mask is beneficial for the removal of acne and dirt that is deeply trapped into the pores. The egg white helps fight the acne problem and the lemon's exfoliating properties help remove acne scars. This is recommended for skin types with acne problems and sensitive type of skin.

Hydrating Papaya Face Mask

Ingredients:

- ½ slice of ripe papaya fruit

- 2 table spoons of yogurt

Instructions:

- Peel and slice the papaya fruit and remove the seeds.

- In a blender, blend the half piece of papaya until the mixture is smooth.

- Add the yogurt and blend until the mixture is thoroughly mixed.

- Pour the mixture into a container and label properly.

Benefits: The papaya facial mask is suitable for sensitive skin since it is made from natural ingredients. The yogurt contains hydrating properties that nourish the skin, and the papaya fruit is a natural exfoliant that whitens the dark spots on the face, making it look more vibrant.

Application of Scrub and Mask

Scrub: To apply the scrub on the face, use gentle circular motions for 3-5 minutes. You can scrub your nose, chin and forehead a little harder. Do not use the scrub on open wounds. To apply the scrub on the body, pay close attention to your hands, feet, knees, and elbows and rub using circular motions for 5-10 minutes. Rinse thoroughly and pat dry the skin with a clean towel.

Mask: Your skin should be cleansed before applying facial mask. It is recommended to open your pores before using the mask. For that, you can take a cloth soaked in tolerable hot water and cover your face with it till it cools down. Then apply a thin layer of mask with your fingers or brush over your face and neck, avoid lips and eyes. Let the mask air dry. It may dry in 10-20 minutes. Relax in the mean time. Remove the mask with a damp sponge or cloth, and then wash your face and pat dry the skin with a clean towel.

Final Words

People with dry skin should not exfoliate as regularly as people with oily skin. Once or twice a week is enough as you do not want to parch your skin. Exfoliation leaves your skin dry and moisturizing is necessary after every exfoliating session. Also, be very careful with the pressure used while exfoliating your face because you do not want to be too harsh on the sensitive skin. Choose your scrub or mask ingredients cautiously, and do proper research about your skin type. Ultimately, gentle and regular exfoliation using natural scrub or mask ingredients would give you smooth and silky skin that feels and looks healthy.

I hope you must have not only enjoyed this book but also tried few recipes for your skin care. If you want to let others know about your experience, please post your valuable and constructive reviews. Your feedback matters and it really does make a difference.

I would greatly appreciate your comment because your review is going to help me improve and update my work. If you found any error or anything you suggest to change or add in this, do let me know at

ypamesh@gmail.com and I promise a quick personal response.

Your review is going to make a true experience for other readers and help them make their buying decision easier. If you'd like to leave a review then all you need to do is go to review section of book and click on "Write a customer review".

CPSIA information can be obtained
at www.ICGtesting.com
Printed in the USA
BVHW041712310820
587706BV00009B/627